The Adventures of BabyBud -An Illustrated Guide to Baby

Contents

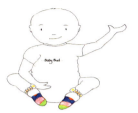

- What is Reflexology?
- About Me
- The Benefits of BabyBuds Baby Reflexology for Baby
- When not to use Baby Reflexology!
- Benefits of Baby Reflexology for Parents
- How to use BabyBuds Guide Book and Preparing for Baby Reflexology
- The Bubbling Spring -The Basic Baby Reflexology Routine
- The Daisy Chain -Sleep ,Calm and Relax Baby Reflexology Routine
- The Whirlpool- Digestion Baby Reflexology Routine
- Big Toe Tree - Wellbeing and Immunity Baby Reflexology Routine
- Foot Diagrams
- Further Information
- Acknowledgements

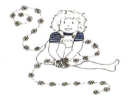

The Adventures of BabyBud - An Illustrated Guide to Baby and Child Reflexology

What is Reflexology?

Reflexology is an ancient holistic healing method that aims to improve health and well-being! The Ancient Egyptians, as early as 2330 B.C, were known to carry out this treatment as can be seen on wall paintings in the Tomb of Ankhmahor.

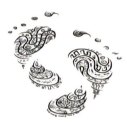

Reflexology is a massage of special reflex points on the feet which act like mirrors reflecting areas of the whole body. Reflexology aims to detect energy blockages which can show themselves as tender or crystal deposits on areas of the foot. These occur in the the part of the foot which relate to the zone of the body which may have an energy imbalance.

The Reflexology Foot Massage technique breaks down these crystals and encourages circulation of blood around the body, promoting self-healing allowing the flow of the body's vital 'Energy'.

Baby Reflexology is based on the same idea as that used in Reflexology for adults, however the Reflexology massage movements on Baby's feet have been adapted in terms of lighter pressures. The length of treatment time is much shorter so as to not to over-stimulate Baby's system.

Baby Reflexology does not replace conventional medicine and if you are at all concerned about the health of your Baby, medical advice must be sought.

Reflexology is an enjoyable relaxing and soothing treatment which is totally natural and may boost immunity and wellbeing for all ages from 4 weeks old to 100+ Years! As BabyBud will show us!

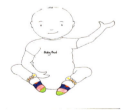

About Me

I am a Reflexologist and Holistic Therapist, gaining my Reflexology Qualification in 2008. I also have a Biomedical Sciences BSc (Hons) Degree and in a previous career have worked in Pathology as a Biomedical Scientist for almost 20 years, which has helped giving me my knowledge of the human body. Very useful to a Reflexologist! I now dedicate all of my time to my interest in the fascinating subject of holistic or complementary therapies, spreading the word of their many benefits.

I have been a firm believer in a holistic approach to health and wellbeing for many years, recognising how, for example, mental stress can cause unwanted and damaging effects on the body.

Reflexology and other holistic therapies aim to achieve a balanced state for the whole body instead of focusing entirely on the symptoms of disease or a physical ailment. The holistic approach aims to balance body and mind before symptoms present themselves and complements conventional medicine.

I provide Reflexology Treatments for adults from my Garden Room at RoseBud Holistics and also I teach BabyBuds Baby Reflexology for Mams and their Babies, teaching BabyBud Baby Reflexology Routines as descibed in this guidebook. These can easily be taught on a one- to- one basis or in small groups which can be a fun and relaxing experience for everyone.

I also have an interest in creative writing,and thus the Adventures of BabyBud were born. The idea of creating a journey around Baby's foot using rhymes and illustration will be exciting and engaging for growing Baby whilst enjoying Baby Reflexology!

I would like to share my passion for Reflexology through the illustrated routines in this Guide Book, with its benefits for improving health and wellbeing of your young family in a totally natural way, while also being exceedingly relaxing! The Routines are suitable for Baby aged from 4 weeks and beyond!

The four simple Routines in this Guide Book follow BabyBud's Adventures using Rhymes to correspond with the special reflexology moves on Baby's feet.

A memorable Journey is created to treasure and the unique bonding experience will be remembered in the years to come. A fun- sharing exerience with family members or siblings or a quiet routine at the end of the day, BabyBuds Baby Reflexology can be taken with you anywhere.

I recommend you try a Reflexology Treatment from a Fully Qualified Reflexologist and experience a blissful hour for yourself in this fast- paced world we live in and just see how you may benefit! Best Wishes,Sarah.

The Benefits of BabyBuds Baby Reflexology for Baby

Baby Reflexology is completely natural, using knowledge of foot maps and gentle pressure of our thumbs and fingers to stimulate the reflex points on Baby's foot which mirrors in Baby's body! Areas in the body may have become imbalanced or Baby maybe experiencing common first year developmental stage symptoms and some relief can be given.

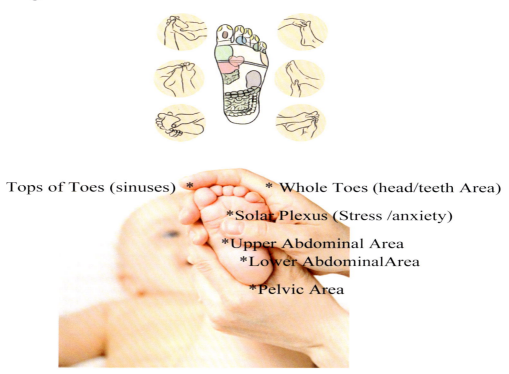

Tops of Toes (sinuses) * * Whole Toes (head/teeth Area)
*Solar Plexus (Stress /anxiety)
*Upper Abdominal Area
*Lower AbdominalArea
*Pelvic Area

Other benefits include addressing feelings of security, non-verbal communication and supporting bonding between Baby and parent!

Baby Reflexology can give some relief from asthma, colic/wind, constipation, diarrhoea, ear ache, eczema, sinus congestion, sleep problems, teething and reflux. Improved general health and wellbeing, relaxation and calmness can be expected also with BabyBuds Baby Reflexology!

BabyBuds Baby reflexology will be fun and enjoyable for both you and Baby and become part of Baby's daily routine, whether on rising, bath time or before bedtime, whenever suits you both best!

The BabyBuds Rhymes which fit with each of the Four Reflexology Routines will become familiar and engage Baby's interest, stimulate speech and imagination, all whilst enjoying the benefits of Reflexology.

When not to use Baby Reflexology!

There are times which are not suitable for Baby to try Reflexology, for example If Baby is feverish, feeling ill or has had their immunisations within 48hrs. If Baby has a skin condition, the massage movements on the foot may spread it further! You know Baby better than anyone in the world, so if baby is unsettled or seems in pain or discomfort then do not go ahead with Baby Reflexology.

If Baby is asleep do not wake them or if Baby seems tired, hungry, crying or pushing away just reassure them and wait until they are happy and rested . Then Baby Reflexology will always be a positive, fun activity for you both!

Benefits of Reflexology for Parents

There are many benefits of Baby Reflexology for you, making the Routines enjoyable for you both! Enjoying time with baby is an empowering experience boosting confidence and supporting bonding between you and Baby.

The moments enjoying reflexology together will become a treasured relaxing interlude whenever you decide to fit it into your daily routine. Dipping into the Guidebook and selecting favourite elements along with BabyBud's Rhyming Adventures as you journey around Baby's foot!

Baby Reflexology can be taken anywhere with you, whether on a train or bus journey or in the supermarket, Baby's feet are quite accessible and for example you will be able to enjoy BabyBud's Daisy Chain Adventure to settle and calm Baby.

How to use BabyBud's Guide Book and Preparing for Baby Reflexology

A warm room without distractions placing baby on their back on a soft mat cocooned by your outstretched legs as you sit on the floor is a good place to begin. Un-fragranced nut free oil such as grape seed or talc free baby powder to hand to use during Baby Reflexology.

Then you must ask Baby Permission and indicate to Baby you are starting, showing baby your hands and rubbing them together so they become familiar with this new experience, sights, sounds and smells!

"Shall we begin BabyBuds Adventures?"

There are only <u>Three Simple massage movements</u> you will use as BabyBud shows you as he ventures around Baby's tiny foot with its different landmarks!

<u>Effleurage</u> which is a stroking or soothing movements with your thumbs you may imagine you are pushing some leaves, as in the rhyme, in an upwards movement across the surface of the foot!

<u>Caterpillar Crawl</u> using your thumb or index finger, inching your way slowly over the surface of the skin using the pad of your thumb or index finger.

<u>Gently pressing then circle movements</u> using the pad of thumb or your index finger in one place or then maybe spirally inwards and outwards, making an imaginary circle bigger then smaller on Baby's foot.

The pressure used is very gentle, not too firm but not so light as to tickle!

I recommend only a few minutes of Baby Reflexology to start with, building up gradually and discovering what works for you and Baby!

There are Four simple Routines, with a BabyBud Adventure to guide you through each. Each one has a unique benefit as well as generally being soothing and relaxing for you both. Also some moves are repeated, allowing you to become familiar with the routines.

The Adventures of BabyBud

The Bubbling Spring

BabyBud BabyBud, where do we go?

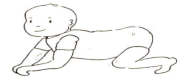

We Creep and Crawl across the Big Toe.

BabyBud BabyBud where shall we go travelling?

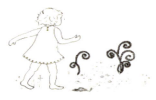

We shall Flow Round and Around the Bubbling Spring,

To Calm and Relax a good Place to Begin!

BabyBud BabyBud, Now where do we go?

Just down this Lane,   March down the Valley,

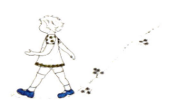
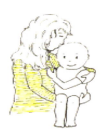

. From Big Toe to Down Low, then back up again

I may need a Carry!

BabyBud BabyBud, Look, See what I've Found! On the Right!
Go up to the Arch, Under the Bridge,

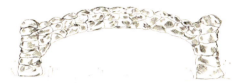

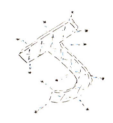

A Jump to the Left, a J made of Crystal, there to be found on the Ground!
BabyBud BabyBud, Now time to relax our lower Back,
Resting heels in our hands,

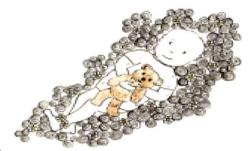

All Calm and Relaxed!

The Adventures of BabyBud
The Daisy Chain

BabyBud BabyBud, Shall we begin Baby Reflex?
At the heel, just hold,

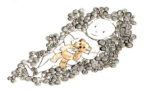

To Calm and Relax our lower backs!

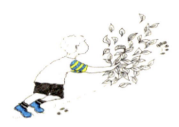

.BabyBud BabyBud,where next do we troop
We shall push some fallen leaves up the steep hill,
From the heel below, collect leaves in a Group!

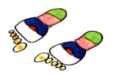

BabyBud BabyBud, Now where do we go?

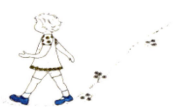

We'll March Down the Valley,
Edge of Big toe to Down Low,
Then Right back up Again,Go,Go,Go!

BabyBud BabyBud,
To Help Clear our snuffly noses!
We'll go Round and Round Toe Tree Tops,

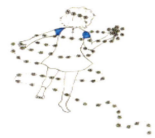

Collecting Daisy Poseys!
BabyBud BabyBud,
Sure to keep your Balance,
Bounce down little toe, with its friend next door,

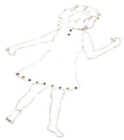

Slowly turn around and around six times in a row!
BabyBud BabyBud,
Gently make me a Daisy chain, to fit around my
Tiny anklet, the softest of Flowers, just like rain!

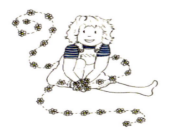

The Adventures of BabyBud
The Whirlpool

BabyBud BabyBud, Where Shall we Start!

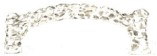

In the Middle, back and forth, under the Arch!
Next BabyBud, we'll jump down from the Arch,

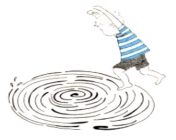

Into the Whirlpool down at the Heel,

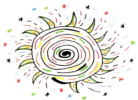

We'll Spin Round and round like a Catherine Wheel!
BabyBud BabyBud, Look see what I've found. On the Right!
Go up to the arch ,under the Bridge,
A Jump to the Left, a J made of Crystal

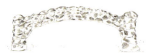

There to be found on the ground!

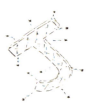

12

On the Right Foot Alone draw a line down from Little Toe,

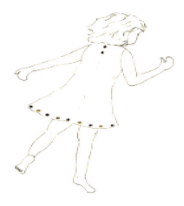

We spin round on the edge,

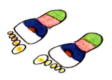

Nearly on our way Home!
To Finish Baby Reflex,
Cup Heels in your Hand,
To Soothe and Calm, Like Warm Soft Sand!

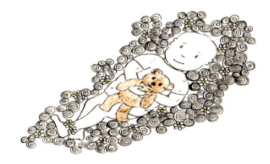

The Adventures of BabyBud

The Big Toe Tree

BabyBud BabyBud, Where shall we go?

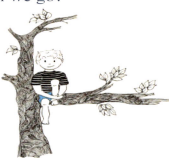

Top of Big Toe Tree ,is a good place to begin,
Look all around in a circle, and down below!
I can hear and see a water slide, between little toe
And the toes nearby,

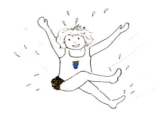

Let's slide down and see,
Weee ,Weeee,Weeee,

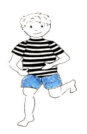
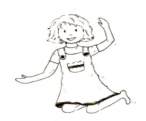

Now Run, Skip and Jump,

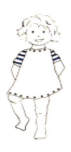

Around Big Toe Tree Trunk.
Next, Into the Whirlpool,

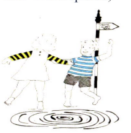

At the bottom of the Tree,
Hold on Tight, as you spin round and round,
Spinning with delight!
To finish our Journey, We shall walk through Toe Trees,

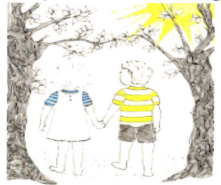

In between the swaying branches,
We watch the sparkling sunshine,
Through leaves rustling in the Breeze.

BabyBuds BubblingSpring! – The Basic Routine

Head Reflex-Move 1
Walk with THUMB across the pad of Big Toe in lines from Top to Bottom 3x. Repeat on front of Big Toe.

Benefits : Pituitary, ear, nose and windpipe

BabyBud BabyBud, where do we go?

We Creep and Crawl across the Big Toe.

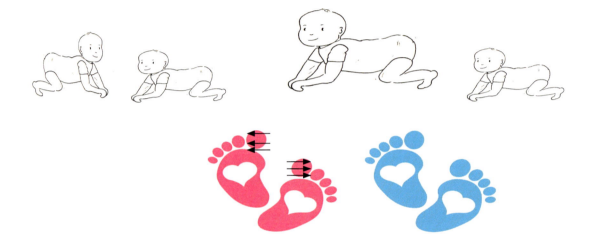

Solar Plexus
Circle in the centre of the Foot just where the arch starts 6X.

Benefits: Helps with anxiety and relaxation

BabyBud BabyBud where shall we go travelling?

We shall Flow Round and Around the Bubbling Spring,

To Calm and Relax a good Place to Begin!

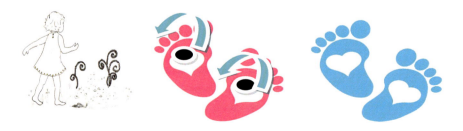

Spine   Using both Thumbs. Walk down the inside edge of each foot from Big Toe to Heel. One Thumb following the other 3X.
Benefits: Spinal nerves & nervous system

BabyBud BabyBud, Now where do we go?

Just down this Lane,   March down the Valley,

From Big Toe to Down Low, then back up again I may need a Carry!

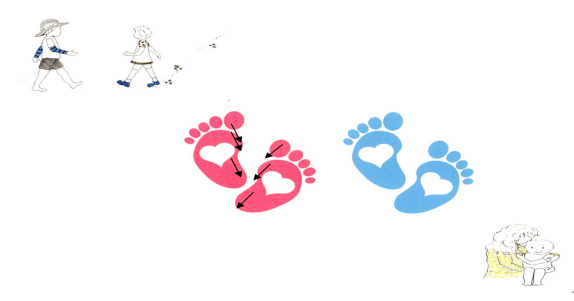

Colon   On the Right Foot, Start from a little way up the heel, thumb walk up side of foot up to middle of foot then thumb walk across middle of foot to other side. 3X On Left. From edge of foot in the middle work across then down edge of foot then flick upwards 3X. **Benefits: Aids digestive system, constipation, diarrohea, wind and stress**

BabyBud BabyBud, Look, See what I've Found! On the Right!

Go up to the Arch, Under the Bridge,

A Jump to the Left, a J made of Crystal, there to be found on the Ground!

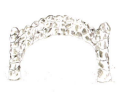 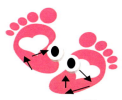 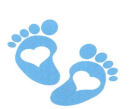 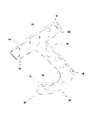

17

Hold the Feet   **Cupping the heels in your hands, helps calm the pelvic area**
Benefits: Pelvic area and lower back

BabyBud BabyBud, Now time to relax our lower Back,

Resting heels in our hands,

All Calm and Relaxed!

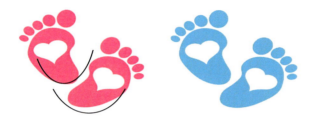

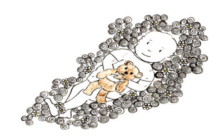

BabyBuds Daisy Chain – Sleep Calm and Relax

Hold the Feet   Take Hold of Baby's Feet. Cupping the heels in your hands, hold for a few seconds while you connect with your baby.

Benefits: Relaxation, communication, bonding

BabyBud BabyBud, Shall we begin Baby Reflex?
At the heel, just hold,
To Calm and Relax our lower backs!

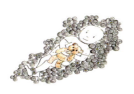 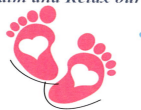 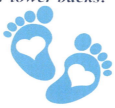

Slide Up   Take hold of baby's feet and using pads of your thumbs slide up the foot from heel to each toe 6X

Benefits: Activates all areas of the body, excellent for calming, soothing and general wellbeing.

BabyBud BabyBud, where next do we troop,
We shall push some fallen leaves up the steep hill,
From the heel below, collect leaves in a Group!

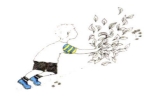 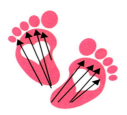 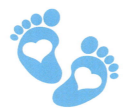

Spine Using two thumbs walk down the side of foot from Big Toe to Heel. Then back to Big Toe 3x

Benefits: stimulates spinal nerves and nervous system.

BabyBud BabyBud, Now where do we go?
We'll March Down the Valley,
Edge of Big toe to Down Low,
Then Right back up Again, Go, Go, Go!

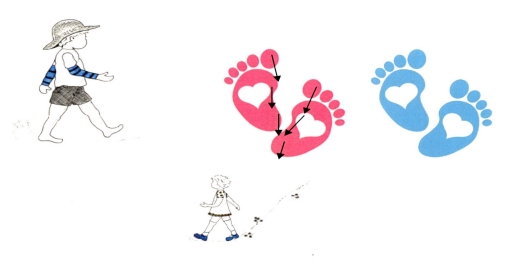

Brain and Sinuses Using the Pads of your Thumbs, gently press into the tops of baby's toes roll in a circular motion, each 6X. **Benefits: Excellent for calming, soothing, relieving head pain, clearing sinuses and general wellbeing.**

BabyBud BabyBud,
To Help Clear our snuffly noses!
We'll go Round and Round Toe Tree Tops,
Collecting Daisy Poseys!
BabyBud BabyBud,
Sure to keep your Balance,

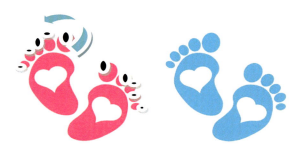
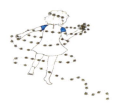

Shoulders and Lungs **Press the pads of your thumb under the Little Toe and 4th Toe in the ball of baby's foot, then do the same under the 3rd and 4th Toe, circle 6X on each area.**

Benefits: Help relax the whole body and create balance

Bounce down little toe, with its friend next door,
Slowly turn around and around six times in a row!

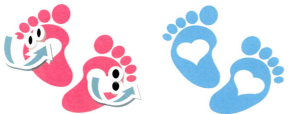
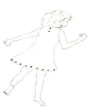

Immune Boost **Hold on to Baby's foot and where the foot meets the leg , using the pads of your fingers or thumbs press gently creating little circles arond the ankle like a bracelet.3X**

Benefits: Calming, soothing and boosting the immune system

BabyBud BabyBud,
Gently make me a Daisy chain, to fit around my
Tiny anklet, the softest of Flowers, just like rain!

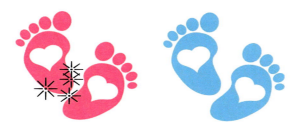
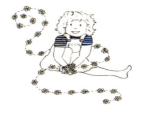

BabyBuds WhirlPool – Digestion

Stomach and Liver Thumb walk gently across the arch of baby's foot in lines 3X.

Benefits: Helps with Digestion and Colic

BabyBud BabyBud, Where Shall we Start!
In the Middle, back and forth, under the Arch!

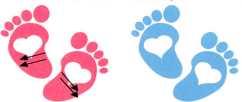 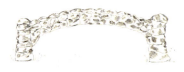

Small intestines and Pelvic area Press and circle into the heel of each foot working in a spiral up to the beginning of the arch, then spiral down to the heel 6X

Benefits::Improves Digestive system, Constipation, Wind and Stress

Next BabyBud, we'll jump down from the Arch,
Into the Whirlpool down at the Heel,
We'll Spin Round and round like a Catherine Wheel!

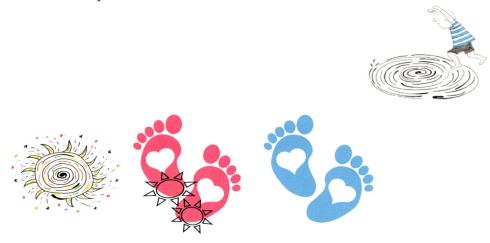

Colon **On the right foot work up and across, then on left foot thumb press across the middle of the foot then down the edge and flick up in a J shape.3X**
Benefits; Improves Digestion, Constipation wind and stress.

BabyBud BabyBud, Look see what I've found. On the Right!
Go up to the arch ,under the Bridge,
A Jump to the Left, a J made of Crystal
There to be found on the ground!

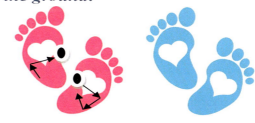

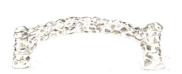 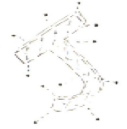

Ileocecal Valve/Appendix **Press with pad of thumb on the right foot only in line with the little toe .Circle 6X.**
Benefits: Prevents backflow of waste solid matter, controls mucous secretions

On the Right Foot Alone draw a line down from Little Toe,
We spin round on the edge,
Nearly on our way Home!

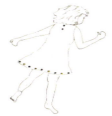 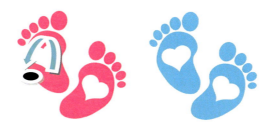

Hold the Feet **Hold onto Baby's feet gently in your Hands**
Benefits: Pelvic and lower back area and Helps Calm Baby

To Finish Baby Reflex,
Cup Heels in your Hand,
To Soothe and Calm, Like Warm Soft Sand!

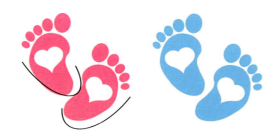

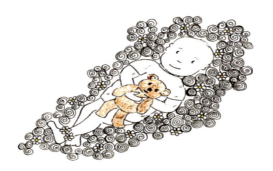

BabyBuds Big Toe Tree – Wellbeing and Immunity

Head – Move 2 Hold Baby's foot and press with the pad of your thumb onto baby's Big Toe and Circle. Repeat circles 3X **Benefits: Brain ,Hypothalamus,pituitary, Mouth and teeth, relaxation, calming, soothing, helps head pains, teething and General wellbeing**.

BabyBud BabyBud, Where shall we go?
Top of Big Toe Tree ,is a good place to begin,
Look all around in a circle, and down below!

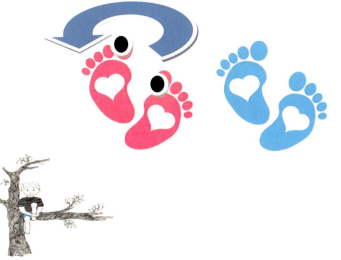

Ears and Eyes With pads of your thumbs slide in between the 5th and 4th toe then press 3X, then slide down in between the 4th and 3rd toe then press 3X. Then rpt by pressing just underneath the toes **Benefits: Ear popping, draining nasal sinuses, balance, calming , soothing, General wellbeing** .

I can hear and see a water slide, between little toe
And the toes nearby,
Let's slide down and see,
Weee ,Weeee,Weeee,

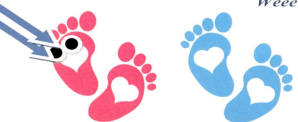
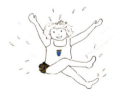

Mouth, Teeth and Nose **Press around the Base of the Big Toe all the way round to the front 3X**
Benefits:.Helps Teething, Breathing and Snuffles

Now Run, Skip and Jump,
Around Big Toe Tree Trunk.

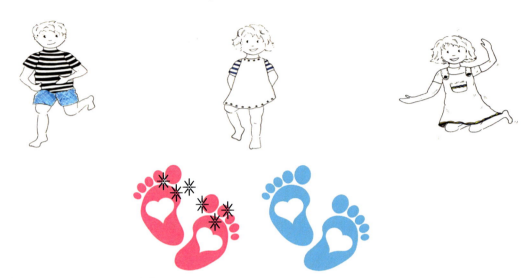

Neck, Thymus and Thyroid **Circle underneath the Big toe and 2nd toe. Big spiral into smaller spiral 3X Benefits: Metabolism, Immunity and strengthens the neck**

Next, Into the Whirlpool,
At the bottom of the Tree,
Hold on Tight, as you spin round and round,
Spinning with delight!

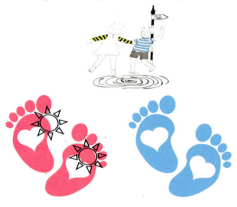

Bronchial and Eustachian **Use your finger to work down the insides of each toe, starting at the Big Toe across to little toe then return. Press at the top and slide down.** **Benefits: Boosts the immunity**

To finish our Journey, We shall walk through Toe Trees,
In between the swaying branches,
We watch the sparkling sunshine,
Through leaves rustling in the Breeze.

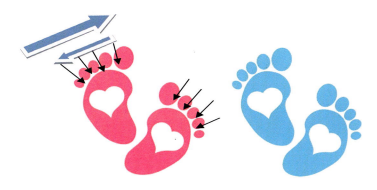

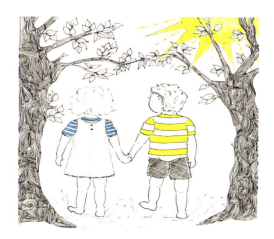

BabyBuds Baby Reflexology Routine Diagrams

Head Reflex 1 *Pituitary, mouth, jaw, ear, nose and windpipe. Repeat 3X*

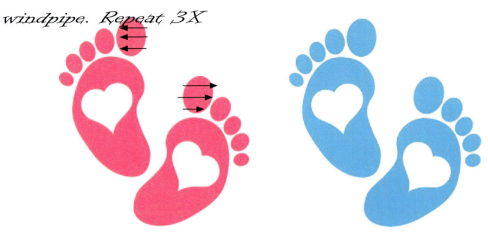

Solar Plexus *Helps with anxiety and relaxes X6*

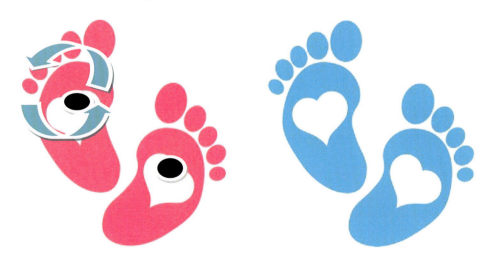

Spine   *Spinal nerves and nervous system x3*

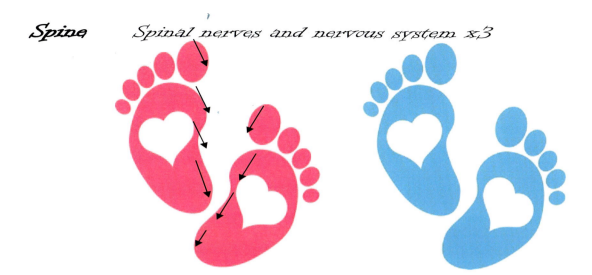

Colon   *Helps Digestion, constipation, wind and Stress*

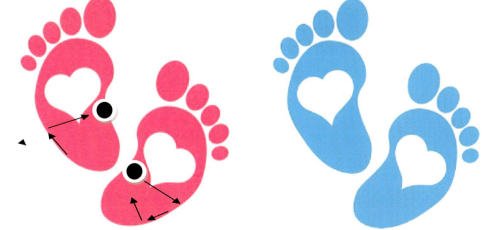

Hold the Feet Relaxation, Communication and Bonding

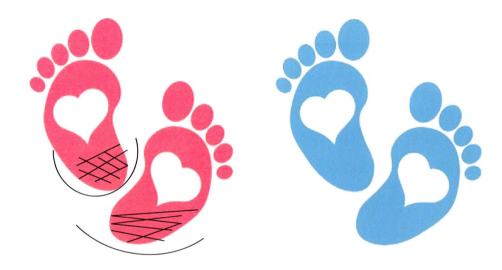

Slide Up Activates all of the body's reflexes, Excellent calming soothing, General wellbeing

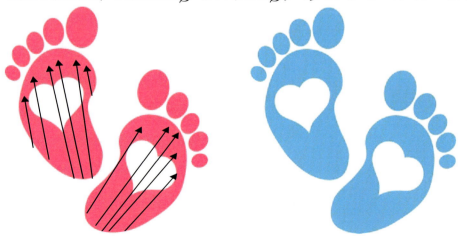

Brain and Sinuses *Head pain, clears sinuses, calming and soothing x6.*

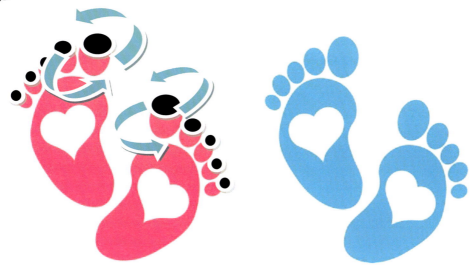

Shoulders & Lungs *Relax the whole body,* **balances** *X6*

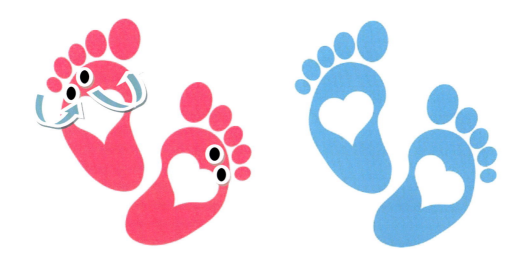

Anklet *Immune Boost x3*

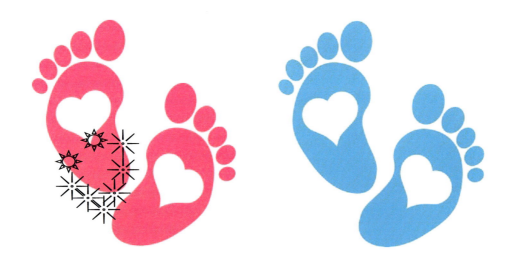

Stomach and Liver *colic and liver x3*

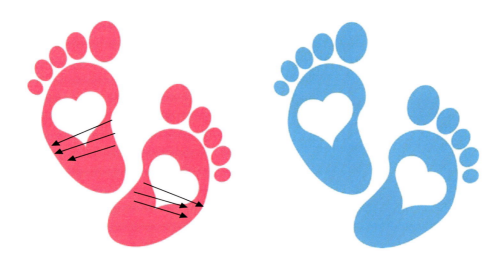

Small Intestines & Pelvic Area Constipation, wind & stress x6

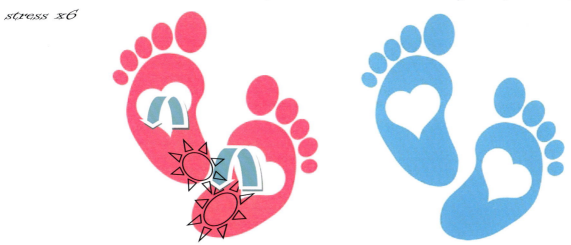

Ileocecal Valve/Appendix controls mucous secretions boosts immunity. X6 **Right Foot only.**

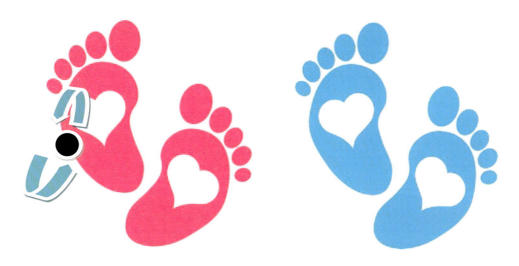

Head Move 2 *Relaxation, teething pain, head pains, calming and soothing. X3*

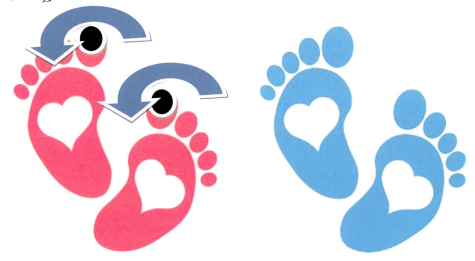

Ears and Eyes *- Balance, ear popping, head pain, calming and soothing.*

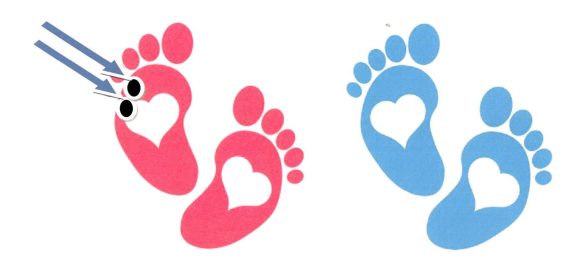

Mouth, Teeth & Nose, Teething, breathing and snuffles x3

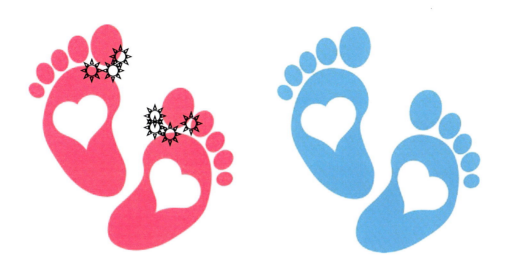

Neck, Thymus and Thyroid - Strengthens the neck, immunity and metabolism

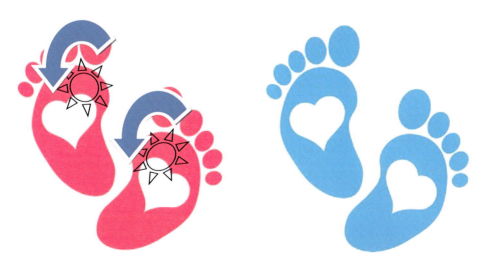

Bronchial & Eustachian — Boosts the Immunity

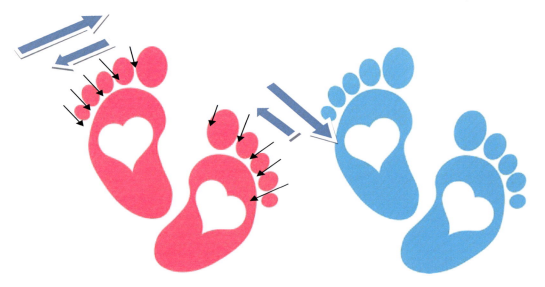

BabyBuds Baby Reflexology Further Information & Resources

RoseBud Holistics, Whitburn ,Sunderland,Tyne and Wear.

Find me on Facebook : RoseBud Holistics

BabyBuds Baby ReflexologyTuition & Mother/Baby Gifts.

Find me on Twitter : sarah@rosebudholistic

I provide BabyBuds Baby Reflexology in the comfort of your own home, one- to-one tuition, or small groups of friends!

Guru Holistic Therapies and Training, GilesGate, Durham,Tyne and Wear.

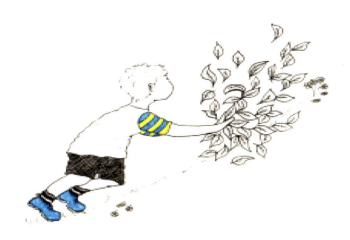

BabyBuds Baby Reflexology Acknowledgements

I would like to give many thanks to my Holistic Therapies Trainer and guide, Ann Ball, of Guru Holistics Therapies and Training, Durham. She has been an invaluable training resource and support, offering an incredible range of holistic therapies including Baby Reflexology Tuition! Many Thanks.

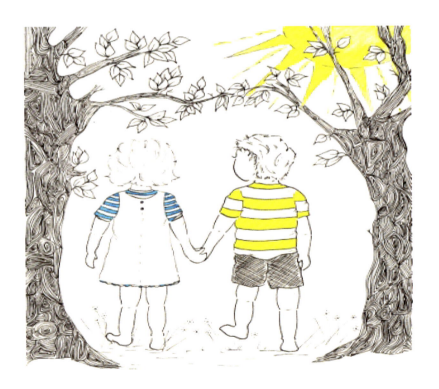